Whole-Body

Health Practices

That Will Change Your Life

Whole-Body Health Practices

That Will Change Your Life

All Natural & Drug Free Remedies for the Mind, Body and Soul

Susanna K. Green

Whole-Body Health Practices That Will Change Your Life

All Natural & Drug Free Remedies for the Mind, Body and Soul

Copyright © 2016 by Susanna K. Green

Book design by Madhouse Design Inc.

Published by Sweet Nectar Publishing

Healthnutsuzy.com

ISBN 978-0-9977022-0-0

I dedicate this book to my husband, Michael. Thank you for loving me the way you do and for sharing your life's journey with me.

Contents

Acknowledgements

Thank you... to all of my family, friends and supporters who love me. I'm so grateful and humbled by the many people I have inspired toward a better life, and will continue to do so.

Wallace King, once again your talent has exceeded my expectations beyond measure; thank you for another amazing book cover creation.

David Winston, thank you for always being willing and ready when I call on you for photos.

Kimberly Kaye of WFKX, thank you for the endorsement and for the amazing radio interviews to help me share my work with the masses.

A special thank you to Iris Holton of the Florida Sentinel Bulletin for the splendid article and endorsement.

Thanks so much to Mikki Val, a remarkable actress whose endorsement means the world to me.

Liana Leal, thank you for the endorsement; you are a remarkable talent at what you do.

Michael Sawyer, my husband, there are so many reasons to thank you; But, in particular, for helping me bring my dreams to fruition.

Laila, my toy poodle, you are the perfect inspiration.

And, as always
Thank you, GOD...

Introduction

From the time of conception, to our teenage years, we were under someone else's authority. We ate what mom cooked and that was that. In our twenties, we were able to explore our true likes and dislikes rather than being told, "Eat your vegetables," that in most cases aren't the most appetizing thing to an adolescent's palate.

I, for one, took my health for granted in my twenties. I ate whatever I wanted, whenever I wanted, without a second thought. I think, I was able to get away with it because I weighed a whopping 98 pounds. I had flat abs and felt great. Even after the birth of my son, Matthew, I somehow reverted right back to my original weight, with no problem. People commented, "You don't look like you've just had a baby." I would venture to say, a lot of us were marred by erratic lifestyle habits in our twenties; we felt invincible.

I was always health conscious but was not consistent in doing what I knew was right to do for my body; like getting more fruits and vegetables into my diet or making sure I stayed hydrated. My fitness routine, was minimal at best and I smoked. It was all about the party scene, drinking myself into a stupor and thinking that's what life was all about. I think, that's the case for a lot of twenty year olds.

When we hit thirty, we become a little more proactive. Our perception matures, allowing us to view life differently, as if we've changed the prescription in our glasses, enabling us to see more clearly. We take life more seriously and value ourselves more. I know I did. I began to feel motivated and passionate about my health, about what I ate and how I treated my body. And, when I hit 40, oh boy, I instinctively understood the true meaning of self-love and what it meant to feel awakened. It was like, a light bulb came on in my head which created epiphanies. The synchronicities were blatant and flowed naturally, until I had no choice but to follow the path that unfolded before me. I finally discovered, how to connect the dots.

I recognized the revelations as a constant flow of gentle nudges, which grew in strength with time, causing me to stop, look and listen; not only with my physical senses but also intuitively, with my spiritual eyes and ears.

As I waited for answers, I continued to explore and learn everything I could, concerning natural ways for people to fuel their bodies with what it needs to heal itself. In my findings, there are six main pillars to being well; nutrition, fitness, weight management, stress management, addiction and emotional health. In my wellness practice, I work specifically in these areas.

I've learned a lot along my health Journey, through study, intuition and trial and error and have made a God-like euphoric discovery that I feel compelled to share with anyone who will listen.

Connecting the mind and body is the missing piece to the puzzle. Many folks have known for centuries that allowing the mind to form a strong alliance with the body is essential for optimal health. Fueling one without the other is detrimental to the entire team.

Introduction

My holistic perspective ties in the wisdom of the East to the science of the West, in which there is no separation of the mind and body. This book is meant to arm you with a plethora of knowledge and empower you to become more conscious of the connection between the mind, body and spirit. Some people will effortlessly understand and some won't. My one and only goal is to lead you to the water, but it's up to you to drink.

Disclaimer

This content is offered on an informational basis only!

No content is intended to be a substitute for professional medical advice, diagnosis or treatment. You should always seek the advice and guidance of a qualified health provider, before:

☆ Making any adjustment to any medication or treatment protocol you are currently using.

☆ Stopping any medication or treatment protocol you are currently using.

☆ Starting any new medication or treatment protocol.

I am not a doctor; I am a wellness coach!

It is very important to note that all of the wellness techniques listed in this book are to enhance health and life force energy only. I do not claim that any of the lifestyle strategies listed here will cure any diseases.

1.

Nutrition

▼

Everything you eat or drink is either fighting disease
or feeding it

As a certified nutrition professional, I am often mistaken for a vegetarian, or vegan. It is a common misconception, that wellness coaches and nutritionists don't eat meat. Well, that is certainly not the case. I don't like labels, but if I had to put one on my personal eating style, it would be closely related to flexitarian. I eat about 20 percent meat and 80 percent whole grains and plant based foods. Also, I avoid processed meat like the plague and opt for meat that has not been modified to extend its shelf life or cured to change the taste.

I help my clients see the benefit in clean, healthy eating habits that will stick for the long-term. If I take away all of the foods they love and enjoy, my programs will not work. It's about building a mindset that promotes the addition of more vegetarian meals, not how many foods I can take away from them. Speaking for myself only, this is my strategy and it works. How do I know? I tested it on myself before trying it on anyone else.

It all started with *Meatless Mondays*. I would prepare my meals as normal, just without the meat. This could include, meatless spaghetti, beans and rice or chicken parmesan, without the chicken. Sometimes, I replaced the chicken with eggplant and discovered, not only how tasty it was but it had a thick texture, very similar to meat. I noticed, I felt satisfied with the replacement.

I must admit, it was quite difficult, at first, trying to come up with meal plans that excluded meat. After having lived in New Orleans for most of my life, preparing a meatless red beans and rice meal was unheard of. But, my determination allowed me to push through. Initially, I thought, "Something is missing." Of course, it was the meat, I missed.

The following Monday came, and it was time to prepare another meatless meal. Again, I was not looking forward to sitting down to a dinner that didn't have one of the main essentials I grew up on and actually loved. Yet again, I pushed through. I experimented, throwing all sorts of ingredients into the pot, with crossed fingers, hoping it would be edible.

The more I prepared these Meatless Monday dinner ideas, the more creative I became. I went online and discovered a whole new world; a world where meatless meals were more prevalent than my mind could fathom. I became obsessed and wanted to try the countless dishes that were vibrantly colored to look absolutely delectable and mouthwatering. So, I taught myself to make many of the vegetarian meals I found on those recipe sites. But, before my exploration and discoveries of the plethora of meatless dishes on the planet, I was stuck in a rut, with only two of my own made-up recipes; whole-grain pasta smothered with raw, fresh vegetables, like onions, garlic, different colored bell peppers, mushrooms and spinach; and my favorite, sautéed kale, caramelized onions and mushrooms over wild rice. Talk about repetitious! Looking back, I realize, it was all part of my health journey, and I embraced not only my new eating style but the entire process, including the growing pains.

I evolved even further, as time went on. Meatless Mondays turned into Vegan Meatless Mondays and then Raw Vegan Meatless Mondays. By slowly weaning myself off meat, I became comfortable enough to go without, completely. By this time, I found myself excited and looking forward to Mondays. I thought in advance, what meal I would make and how good it would taste. I relished at the opportunity to learn as many recipes as I could. I set goals for myself to eat nine servings of fruits and vegetables in a day and was super excited about reaching my goal.

My thoughts were not on the fact that meat had been omitted but that I was doing something so wonderful for my body, by adding all of the different types of fruits and vegetables. I didn't even realize, I had changed my mindset. It was automatic. I allowed the belief that eating healthy would give me longevity and a good quality of life, which shaped my thoughts about how I thought about food, which governed my actions to make all of those healthy, delicious meals.

I was thrilled to discover a whole new world and began my excursion deeper down the rabbit hole. What was so elating to me was, I found myself implementing veggies that I had never eaten before, like zucchini, spaghetti squash and watercress.

I could now enjoy avocado, lightly sprinkled with sea salt; a plate of nuts and berries; celery sticks dipped in homemade Pico de gallo salsa, red, orange and yellow bell peppers dipped in guacamole and of course, different types of salads without giving meat a second thought.

Now that I had Mondays securely tucked under my belt, I was able to decrease my meat intake on a regular basis, sometimes for 30 days at a time. After sampling the different styles of eating, I was capable of making an educated decision on what nutrition style would be best for me.

Although, the transition was not easy, at first, it became easier, the more I practiced. I learned a lot by trial and error, as with any new project that is learned from scratch. Sometimes, I was uncomfortable and felt like a fish out of water, but I made it...I made it!

Ask yourself this question…

Every time I put anything into my mouth, food or drink, "am I fighting disease or feeding it?"

This will help you to be conscious of everything that goes into your body, good or bad.

1. What is conscious eating?

Conscious eating is eating with intention while paying attention

Aside from chewing your food 32 times and eating slowly without distraction, conscious or mindful eating encompasses the entire process of eating:

- Being conscious of how food makes you feel, physically and emotionally
- Savoring each specific taste

- Allowing yourself to feel pleasant sensory responses
- Trusting your inner wisdom to guide the entire process
- Intuitively knowing how much to eat to feel content
- Using all your senses when choosing, preparing and eating food
- Create a sacred atmosphere to enjoy your meals
- Simply ask yourself (close your eyes, take deep breaths, place your hands on your abdomen and ask, "What do you need?)
- Being aware of physical hunger opposed to physiological hunger

2. *Physical Hunger v's Physiological Hunger*

a. Physical hunger

- Builds gradually
- Feels satisfied with any food
- Causes satisfaction, not guilt
- Occurs several hours after meal
- Once full, you can stop eating

b. Physiological Hunger (emotional, mental, stress or boredom eating)

- Develops suddenly and feels urgent
- Craves specific comfort foods that persists, even when full
- Triggers guilt and shame
- Has no timeframe
- Causes gluttony

3. Nutrition Health Practices

a. Stay hydrated

The human body is made up of over 70% water. Staying hydrated has major health benefits like better muscle function, joint and brain protection, digestion, mood and even improved immune health. Drink filtered water or find a spring nearest you, which is living water. Drinking living water is a major factor in health.

b. Drink warm liquids with your meal

For digestive health and to reduce metabolic waste, drinking water at room temperature opposed to cold, especially in the morning and with a meal is key. And, for an added punch, add lemon.

c. Eat only what you need

Your body is intelligent and knows exactly what it needs to run efficiently. Eat when you are physically hungry, but do not mistake hunger for thirst. Try drinking a glass of water first, to see if it curbs your appetite. If you are truly hungry, eat slowly so that you're able to recognize when you feel satisfied and then put the fork down. Eat only until satisfied, not full.

d. Have Meatless Mondays

Meat is the culprit for many health problems in today's world, especially processed meat which contain nitrates. Aside from the filthy living conditions and close quarters animals endure, they are often beaten, electrocuted and fed a genetically modified diet. They are pumped full of drugs and are diseased by the time they are killed.

Set aside one day of the week to start the weaning process, taking you from a large meat consumption to a moderate amount and then less and less, until you are down to eating meat once or twice a week. If you must eat meat regularly, choose unprocessed meat that has not been modified to extend its shelf life or change its taste.

Try fasting from meat for 30 days, every six months to cleanse your body from carcinogens.

e. Organic when possible

Conventional farmers use pesticides, synthetics and other dangerous chemicals to protect their crops from pests. This can be damaging to your health. Organic produce and other foods are pricy but are not covered in toxic substances that can cause serious health issues.

f. Incorporate raw nuts and seeds into your diet

Both nuts and seeds are a great natural source of vitamins, minerals, protein, healthy fat, and dietary fiber, which can help reduce levels of inflammation and protect against cardiovascular disease. They can stabilize your blood sugar levels and improve cholesterol and reduce your risk of type 2 diabetes.

Most nuts, are high in calories. So, eating the recommended standard serving size is key to maintaining a healthy weight. Eat 1 ½ ounces of nuts per day which roughly equals 1/3 cup. When eating nuts or seeds for the first time, beware of any nut allergies. Tree nuts are one of the food allergens most often linked to anaphylaxis.

My top five healthiest nuts:

- Walnuts
- Almonds
- Macadamia nuts
- Brazil Nuts
- Pecans

My top five healthiest seeds:

- Sunflower seeds
- Hemp seeds
- Chia seeds
- Flax seeds
- Pumpkin seeds

g. Enjoy a vegetable juice/smoothie everyday

One of the major benefits of vegetable smoothies is that they allow you to consume several servings of vegetables in one sitting. Vegetables are extremely nutrient-dense and full of fiber.

Strive for 2-4 servings of fruit a day and 4-5 servings of vegetables for a total of 9 servings of fruit and vegetables, every day.

h. Limit sugar intake

Buy unsweetened food or drink products!

- Once you know where sugar hides, you can start making changes

- Buy foods labeled, no added sugar or unsweetened

Don't go cold turkey

Cut back slowly!

- Example#1- If you normally put two packets of sugar in your coffee, for instance, try one for a week, then half, and finally add only a splash of milk.
- Example#2- For your yogurt, mix half a serving of sweetened yogurt with half a serving of plain, and eventually move on to adding natural sweetness with fresh fruit.

Never eat artificial sugar
When reducing sugar intake, you may be tempted to switch to artificial sugars for your sweet fix. But, resist reaching for the diet soda, sugar-free candy and packets of artificial sugar in your latte. When you eat something sweet, your body expects calories and nutrition, but artificial sugars don't give your body those things.

Don't drink it
Avoiding soda is a good idea. Even drinks that are considered healthy can contain more of the sweet stuff than you're supposed to have in an entire day.

- Enhanced waters (eight teaspoons per bottle)
- Bottled iced teas (more than nine teaspoons per bottle)
- Energy drinks (almost seven teaspoons per can)
- Bottled coffee drinks (eight teaspoons per bottle)
- Store-bought smoothies (more than a dozen teaspoons for a small size)

Add more flavor

- Use vanilla bean and vanilla extract, spices, and citrus zests to add sweetness to foods without having to use sugar, and for zero calories.
- Order an unsweetened latte and add flavor with cocoa or vanilla powder
- Skip the flavored oatmeal and add a sweet kick with cinnamon, nutmeg and ginger.

To cut down on sugar, you should read the nutrition facts label on all products you purchase. The nutrition facts label tells you how many grams of sugar is in each serving. The World Health Organization Guidelines recommend only 25 grams of sugar per day. That's 10 grams less than amount found in sodas. A 12 ounce can of cola has 35 grams of sugar, which is 10 grams over the allowance.

Track your sugar intake

Check the labels of all packaged foods that you eat. If you're taking in more sugar than you mean to, take a look at where the sugar in your diet comes from and you might see some obvious ways to cut back. For example, just trading in that afternoon cola for an unsweetened iced tea could cut 50 grams of added sugar out of your diet in a single swipe. If you eat out, you can often get detailed nutrition information on restaurant websites. Don't worry about the natural sugar in fresh fruit or unsweetened dairy products, but make sure to count any sugar that you put into your coffee or honey that you drizzle over your oatmeal.

Learn sugar aliases
When you read food labels, you'll need to look for more than just the word, *sugar.* Sugar hides under several sneaky names, including, brown sugar, corn sweetener, corn syrup, fruit juice concentrates, high fructose corn syrup, honey, invert sugar, malt sugar, molasses, raw sugar, sugar molecules ending in 'ose' (dextrose, fructose, glucose, lactose, maltose, sucrose).

i. Drink green tea

Green tea has many amazing properties that can keep you in tip-top shape. It is full of powerful antioxidants and can kill bacteria or at the very least, inhibit their growth. This tea kills free radicals that wreak havoc on normal cells in the body, causing you to age quicker as well as normal cell growth that can lead to cancer.

j. Eat foods that are high in phytochemicals (chemicals from the energy of the sun)

Eat foods that are the colors of the rainbow and foods that have the six tastes of life: sweet, sour, salty, pungent, bitter, and astringent.

4. How to choose your best eating style

Dieting is counterproductive and can do damage to your metabolism. It is more times than not, a temporary fix. I personally prefer not to use the restrictive measures of following a specific diet plan, but many people welcome the structure.

My successful nutrition strategy is simple; eat whole, nutrient-dense foods.

- Whole foods-Unprocessed foods that are free from additives and artificial substances.
- Nutrient-dense foods-Foods full of nutrients but relatively low in calories.

a. Listen to biofeedback

Notice how you feel after a meal. Do you feel, bloated, flatulent or uncomfortable in anyway? Notice your energy level, mood, appetite, bowel movements and sleep patterns. If these things are off, it can be signs of the food not being in agreement with you.

Pay attention to how each meal affects you, physically, as well as mentally; grade your symptoms from mild to severe. Keep a journal for this sole purpose, and use it every day as a guide. By doing this, you may uncover food allergens and other culprits making you sick.

b. Identify food allergies

There are eight common food allergens and over 150 uncommon. It is essential to listen to your body when choosing a diet.

The BIG 8 allergenic foods:

- Milk
- Eggs
- Fish
- Wheat
- Crustacean shellfish
- Soy
- Tree nuts

- Peanuts

c. Consider medical conditions

There are tons of diet plans to choose from, but finding the one that caters to your specific ailment is key. Such as, *The Fertility Diet,* which increases ovulation and helps you get pregnant faster.

d. Best suits your lifestyle

When searching around for the perfect nutrition strategy, you must take several key things into consideration; your budget, any health conditions, which friends you'll choose to support you through this time of transition and an iron clad line of attack to keep you disciplined.

e. Have definite goals

Put together a clear strategy of what you want to do. Be specific. Write your plan down on paper to refer back to as needed. Measure your goals to keep track of your progress. Set attainable goals that are realistic for you to achieve. Pick a timeframe to reach your goal. Upon achieving your goal, don't forget to reward yourself for a job well done.

5. Fasting

Fasting is the ideal remedy for our typical overindulgences. There's nothing wrong with enjoying our food, but excess food on a continuous basis creates a burden for the body. When it has to handle more than what's needed, it suffers. Imagine at work how you feel, when you're handed a huge workload; more than what you can handle in your eight hour day, more than what is comfortable for you. You're under pressure, but you have to manage somehow. So, you attend to the most important matters first and set aside those that can wait for later. This is what our bodies do when they're overworked. They tend to tuck things away for another day; whatever task can be postponed, will be. And, more work is dumped on them at every meal or snack time, whether they're ready or not. This is why fasting is a beautiful gift that you can give to yourself. It's a vacation for your weary overworked, underappreciated body.

During a fast, energy is diverted away from the digestive system when it's not in use and it's redirected toward the metabolism and immune system. All fasts will cleanse and detoxify your mind, body and soul. Even just intermittent, short fasts will reward you with many wonderful benefits.

7 main benefits of fasting are:

- Rest the digestive system:
  Fasting allows your digestive system a break, so your organs don't have to work so hard.
- Cleanse and detoxify the body:
  When we eat food that is unhealthy, toxins get into our bodies and when we fast from those foods, the body has less junk to pump out.
- Create a break in eating patterns:
  Who doesn't love to be able to take some time off from work and go on a restful vacation once in a while? That's what fasting does for your body, allows it to rest.
- Promote greater mental clarity:

When our gut is in disarray, so is the rest of our body. Toxins run amuck inside our bodies, wreaking havoc, on our physical, mental and emotional well-being.

- Cleanse and heal *stuck* emotional patterns:
During a fast, toxic junk is removed from the body. We tend to think more clearly and upon doing so, negative thoughts and feelings are brought to the surface and can be more readily identified as toxic thoughts, which is a good thing. Now that you have confronted your inner demons, they must flee.
- Lead to a feeling of physical lightness and increased energy levels:
Eliminating toxins will free up a lot of your energy, leaving you feeling light as a feather.
- Promote an inner stillness, enhancing spiritual connection:
If you want a deeper connection with God and/or your higher self, do a fast while meditating and praying to quiet your spirit and open your spiritual eyes to see and your spiritual ears to hear from within. Particularly, things that you need to know to light your path as you continue on your journey in this life.

Physical, Mental/Emotional and Spiritual conditions improved from fasting

a. Physical benefits: Fasting is called *The Miracle Cure* because the list of physical conditions improved are long and varied:

- Allergies
- Arthritis
- Digestive disorders

23

- Skin conditions
- Cardiovascular disease
- Asthma

b. Mental/Emotional benefits: Fasting allows you to see things clearly, from a more appropriate perspective. You may experience:

- A lift from depression
- Improved concentration
- Less anxiety
- Sleeping better, waking more refreshed

c. Spiritual benefits: Through fasting and prayer together, the Holy Spirit can transform your life. Fasting enables the Holy Spirit to reveal your true spiritual condition, resulting in repentance, and a transformed life.

Types of fasts:

a. Dry fasting: Also known as Absolute Fast, Black Fast and Hebrew Fast. This type of fast is the most extreme of all fasts. It has spiritual roots and consists of foregoing food for short to long periods of time.

- Hard dry fasting: Hard dry fasting is when you avoid all contact with water; no baths or showers, no brushing teeth, washing hands or face, washing dishes and so on. Water does not touch your body at all!
- Soft dry fasting: Soft dry fasting restricts you from drinking water, but you can bathe and allow water to touch the outer portions of your body.

b. Liquid fasting: Liquid fasting means the abstaining from all solid foods—only liquids are ingested. It delivers the greatest health benefits physically in the shortest period of time. Detox will occur more quickly than other types of fasts.

- Water fasting: The simplest and oldest form of liquid fasting.
- Juice fasting: Juice fasting offers lots of nutritional support in a pure and natural form. Almost any fruit or vegetable can be juiced.
- Master cleanse: (aka Lemonade diet)
- The master cleanse is for intestinal cleansing, claiming you'll drop pounds, detox your digestive system and feel very energetic. It consists of three things: Morning salt water flush, 6 to 12 ten ounce glasses of master cleanse lemonade mixture and a nightly herbal laxative tea.

c. Partial fasting: With partial fasting, detoxing will be a little slower but is a great way to start if you are a beginner.

6. Which diet is the best one?

The Paleo diet may be best, if you have an autoimmune disease or digestive disorders. It's also a great diet for those who want to manage their weight. The Paleo diet emphasizes wild-caught meat and fish with plenty of fruits and vegetables but does not include grains, legumes or dairy.

The Mediterranean diet may be best if you are looking to combat inflammation. It can also reduce your risk of heart attack and stroke. This diet is a plant based, whole-food diet, including, fresh fruits and vegetables, whole grains, legumes, olive oil, nuts and red wine; smaller amounts of fish, eggs, chicken, full-fat dairy and very little red meat.

The DASH diet- DASH stands for Dietary Approach to Stop Hypertension. If you suffer from high blood pressure, eating according to this diet may be the way to go.

The MIND diet is the hybrid of both the DASH and Mediterranean diets. It may prevent Alzheimer's disease with brain-healthy foods that are rich in vegetables, whole grains, berries and nuts.

The Mayo clinic diet was designed for people with prediabetes and type 2 diabetes by lowering blood sugar and keeping levels stable; emphasizing fruits, vegetables and whole grains.

As you can see, there are many diet plans on the market that cater to specific ailments and health conditions. This can be good if you are working toward a specific goal, to combat a particular ailment. If you just want to eat healthy, in general, you can't go wrong by eating a whole, plant based diet.

Colors to eat to nourish you

Example: If you have a lung condition such as asthma, eat white colored foods, like cauliflower. If you have rheumatoid arthritis, eat orange colored foods, such as apricots or oranges.

- **Red-** Blood building, heart strengthening
- **Orange-** Anti-inflammatory
- **Yellow-** Tissue repair
- **Green-** Neutralizer, deodorizer, liver detoxifier
- **Blue-** Stem cells, bone marrow, creativity, throat, thyroid

- **Purple**- Central nervous system protector, brain, eyes
- **Brown**- Intestines, digestive tract
- **White**- Beneficial to the lungs
- **Black**- Jing; primordial life force essence; longevity; marrow

Juicing v's Smoothie

If you are just getting started on your health journey, the first place to start is to begin juicing. Juice every morning on an empty stomach with one cup of fresh, organic juice. Use lighter vegetable types, like cucumber, carrots and celery. As you evolve, you can move up to the heavier green vegetables, like kale. In the beginning, your body needs to get adjusted to all of the *real food* it will be getting. You will begin to detox. After about a month, slowly implement drinking smoothies. Smoothies are full of fiber; juicing leaves the pulp behind and extracts the fiber. Notice your eliminations and how much fiber your body can handle. Tweak your recipes to suit your body's specific needs.

Vegetable Juice recipe (beginners)

1 cucumber
2 celery stalks
1 carrot
1 lemon (unpeeled)

Vegetable juice recipe (advanced)

8 large leaves of kale with stem
½ inch knob of ginger (peeled)
1 beet root
¼ green pepper
½ inch knob of turmeric (peeled)

2.

Fitness

▼

The body achieves what the mind believes

Have you tried to lose weight and haven't been successful, after trying everything, from cutting out certain foods, going to the gym and even taking weight loss supplements to suppress your appetite?

I hear this a lot in my business. I ask my clients' one simple question, "Do you truly believe, without a shadow of a doubt, you can achieve your desired results?"

I'm often met with a perplexed look. As if, they are wondering why I'm asking such a ridiculous question. I often ask because people are not connecting their mind and body to help meet their hearts desire. If it is your aspiration to lose 20 pounds, you must believe that you can. Speak positive words aloud, so your ears hear what your mouth says and relay those messages to your brain which will then get your body ready for the task ahead. You will find yourself to be more motivated than before and begin to actually enjoy the process of working toward your goal. Exercise won't feel like such a daunting task. You'll find ways of making time for it, even if that means in small intervals, throughout the day.

I am one of those people who does not like going to the gym. I do not feel comfortable working out around crowds of people, nor do I like them watching me. I don't like wiping off other folks' sweat from the machines and constantly having to sanitize my hands. I'm a medium-grade germophobe.

I tried, time and time again, buying multiple gym memberships throughout my life, until, one day, it hit me. Going to the gym is just not for me. I realized, I love the outdoors, being in nature. I absolutely feel amazing walking through the park or a hiking trail. I love to be near water, taking in the scenery of God's green earth that he so impeccably constructed. I love to bask in the fresh air and listen to the subtle sounds in the background while the sun provides my body with vitamin D. I appreciate the whole experience.

I wondered why I just could not get motivated and was full of excuses as to why I couldn't get to the gym. I became annoyed with myself for wasting money and being stuck in contracts that I couldn't get out of. But, I forced myself to go anyway. While I was there, I was not my best self. I didn't feel joy in my heart or a quietness in my spirit. I was riddled with anxiety that staggered me, nonetheless, I pushed myself because I'm not a quitter.

It wasn't until I found something I truly enjoyed, that I was able to get my desired results. Instead of me briskly walking on the treadmill, I briskly walked, did squats, and lunges through the park trails. I've since added many other therapies to my morning exercise routine; rebounding, inversion therapy, massage chair therapy, earthing, stretching and aqua yoga.

Just as the gym is not my thing, being in nature may not be your thing. It may be too hot, too quiet or too uninteresting. You may need the excitement of seeing and being seen or interacting with other people.

The point is, find what will make you grow younger, become happier and live longer. It's different for everyone. Just make sure you get your fitness in daily, somehow.

You can just about imagine all of the many excuses I've heard, as to why people don't exercise.

Here are a few:

> *"It's so hard to fit exercise into my schedule; my kids keep me so busy."*
>
> *"I can't find anyone to go with me; I can't go by myself, I need an exercise partner."*
>
> *"I hate going to the gym, where people can watch me exercise."*
>
> *"I'm too fat to go to the beach and swim in the ocean!"*
>
> *"I can't take long walks: my feet hurt."*
>
> *"My back hurts and I have arthritis."*
>
> *"I don't need to exercise: I eat right."*
>
> *"I've never exercised before; now, I'm too old."*

To my skeptics and naysayers...

If you've tried everything else which has not yielded your desired results, could it hurt to add some positive expressions to your lifestyle? Don't knock it until you've tried it, yourself.

And, for those of you who think you're too old, too fat, too bald, too crippled, with one foot in the grave or just too lazy to exercise; stop making excuses and get over it!

If you don't like the gym, get out in nature. If you don't like nature, go to the gym. If you don't like either, get an exercise DVD and get moving in the comfort of your own home. Whatever you decide to do, do it with positive intentions and desires. Speak positive words that you truly believe... Proclaim it! It's best to make up your own statements, but here are a few positive affirmations I came up with to get you started:

"I'm so excited to take this walk today; I know I'm going to shed some of this stubborn belly fat."

"I know these pounds are going to fall right off."

"I know with every step I take today, my health will improve."

"I'm going to be so sexy this summer at the beach."

"Once I get moving, I know I'm going to feel great!"

Exercise and physical activity are a great way to feel better, gain health benefits and have fun, all at the same time. It can help prevent excess weight gain or help maintain weight loss. When you engage in physical activity you burn calories. The more intense the activity, the more calories you burn.

Regular physical activity can improve your muscle strength and boost your endurance. Exercise and physical activity deliver oxygen and nutrients to your tissues and help your cardiovascular system work more efficiently. When your heart and lungs work more efficiently, you have more energy. You can be so much more productive in your day when you feel energized, which may have a positive effect on your sex life and in other areas, too. Men who exercise regularly are less likely to have problems with erectile dysfunction than men who don't. Women who regularly exercise may experience enhanced arousal.

Mild to moderate intensity aerobic activity is enough to change your life for the better, but moderate to vigorous activity can double those benefits.

- Moderate amount of activity (2 ½ hours a week)
- Vigorous amount of activity (1 ¼ hours a week)

Exercise is a very important piece to the puzzle in order to live your best quality life.

Why exercise is important:

- It gets your blood flowing
- Allows lymph to flow normally
- Increases circulation
- Boosts energy
- Combats medical conditions
- Reduces stress
- Regulates weight
- Helps control addictions
- Improves mood

Exercise is as good for the mind as it is the body, not only for improving physical functioning, but it also helps your brain process information better. It can be as effective as antidepressant medication at relieving depression and improving mood. It can help you to control your appetite, lose weight, shed inches and lower your risk for a variety of serious diseases. Regular physical activity can help you fall asleep faster and even deepen your sleep.

As a general goal, aim for at least 30 minutes of physical activity a day. Mixing up different types of exercise can add variety to your workouts and broaden the health benefits. While any kind of exercise offers tremendous health benefits, different types of exercise focus more on certain aspects of your health.

The key to success in fitness is finding a physical activity that you love and just do it. Take your time and try a few different ones to see which one you can commit to. If you get bored, try something new.

3 main exercise types:

- Aerobic fitness: Increases the amount of oxygen that goes to the heart and muscles, which strengthens your heart and increases endurance.
- Strength training: Weight lifting or resistance training builds muscle and bone mass, improves balance and prevents falls. It's one of the best counters to frailty in old age.
- Flexibility exercises: Stretching, qigong, tai chi and yoga help prevent injury, enhance range of motion, reduce stiffness and limit aches and pains.

1. Holistic ways to get fit

a. Walk 10,000 steps everyday

To maintain normal health, 6000 steps per day will suffice. To lose weight, walk 10,000 steps per day.

Walking every day will:

- Strengthen your heart
- Lower the risk of disease
- Help prevent dementia
- Keep your weight in check
- Give you energy

And if you walk on a beautiful sunny day, it'll increase your vitamin D levels.

Exercise can help you:

- Relieve stress and anxiety
- Improve self esteem
- Sleep well
- Cope with life

b. Walk briskly

Brisk walking requires you to take 120 steps per minute.

Other moderate aerobic activities:

- Cycle briskly (10 to 12 miles per hour)
- Swimming
- Take a dance class
- Playing golf
- Sailing
- Shoot baskets
- Mow the lawn with walking mower
- Sweep, mop or vacuum
- Hula Hoop
- Do crunches

- Walk up and down stairs

Other vigorous aerobic activities:

- Jogging
- Hit the hiking trails
- Cycling (12 mph or more)
- Carry heavy loads (moving furniture)
- Join a soccer team
- Cross country skiing
- Swimming fast
- Play a game of basketball, football or volleyball

c. Stretch

As you age, your muscles stiffen. Range of motion in the joints can become weakened. Better flexibility can improve your performance in physical activities or decrease your threat of injuries by supporting your joints through their full range of motion, enabling your muscles to work most efficiently.

There are two main types of stretching:

- Dynamic stretching (pre-workout): This method involves motion and ramps up the nervous system, putting your body through its full range of motion.
- Static stretching (mid and post workout): This method involves no motion and dulls the nervous system. This is the typical *stretch and hold* technique.

  Health benefits of stretching:

- Pain relief

- Reduced muscle tension
- Increased energy levels
- Increased range of motion in the joints
- Increased blood flow to the muscles
- Relaxation and stress relief
- Enhanced muscular coordination
- Improved posture

d. Do Qigong

Qigong, an ancient Chinese discipline, involving slow meditative body movements that integrates physical postures, focused attention and breathing techniques. This form of martial arts is highly regarded as an extremely effective health care system that has many health benefits.

e. Do Tai Chi

Tai Chi, a type of martial arts, which originated from Qigong. It is known for its defense techniques and has an array of health benefits, including alleviating anxiety and stress. Tai Chi has multiple low-impact styles. It does not have need of any special equipment nor require much space.

f. Have sex

Having sex counts as moderately intense exercise, helping to boost your heart rate, strengthen muscles and burn calories. Men burn approximately four calories per minute and women burn roughly three calories per minute. It can even help you maintain balance and flexibility.

g. Sit less...Move more

Sitting is now thought of as the new smoking and can have serious health risks for the short and long-term. It is considered sedentary behavior and can shorten your life, particularly from heart disease. Keep in mind, you may be getting enough exercise but that does not mean you still aren't sitting too much. As a general rule, try not to sit any longer than three hours a day.

Tips to sit less:

- When watching TV, get up and walk during commercials
- Take the stairs instead of the elevator or escalator
- Park as far away from work or the grocery store as you can
- Take a break from your computer every 30 minutes

h. Get inverted

Inverting has many physical, mental and cosmetic health benefits from improving circulation and lung function to decreasing physical pain and relieving stress. Inversion is excellent at improving lymphatic system function and the anti-aging effects are a nice bonus.

i. Use a rebounder

Rebounding on a mini trampoline is ideal to work every cell in your body. It's a unique way to exercise, using the forces of acceleration and deceleration. It's great for detoxifying and giving you an immunity boost. It is an effective lymphatic drainage booster. Most people don't realize the lymph in their bodies have become stagnant due to toxic waste overload. Using a re-bounder for just ten minutes a day is beneficial for your skeletal system and it increases cell energy.

j. Do yoga

Yoga is recognized as one of the most healthy, balanced forms of exercise in the world. It's all about harmonizing the mind with the body, involving various breathing techniques, yoga postures and meditations. Yoga creates balance in the body through developing both flexibility and strength.

Pre-Workout Juice Recipe

3 Carrots (large)
1 clove garlic
1 Cantaloupe (small)

Post-Workout Juice Recipe

1 cup blueberries
1 cup grapes (red)
3 celery stalks
1 beet root

3.

Weight Management

▼

Diets are temporary; healthy lifestyle changes are permanent

In my coaching practice, I am often asked, which diet is the best one for losing weight? My answer is, "it's different for everyone." No two people are genetically alike, and we all have different medical conditions and even diverse food preferences. Therefore, In order to be successful at losing weight, you need a strategy that fits your lifestyle, doesn't require you to eat things you don't like and give up all the foods you do like.

When I turned 40, I noticed how my metabolism began to slow down. I was never a dieter, per se, just tried to make healthy food choices. But, there was one food that had a serious hold on me. I had been a devout bread eater with reckless abandon, all my life. This bread-eating trait runs in my family. I've always loved bread of all types, Italian bread, French bread, croissants, bagels, crackers, pita wraps, biscuits, pancakes, pizza, doughnuts, warm, gooey pretzels from the kiosk at the mall...you name it. If it was made from dough, I ate it.

One day, my precious poodle, Laila and I, were out on a walk and a neighbor stopped me to chit chat, as he usually did. I have to admit, it was a little annoying that my exercise routine had to come to a screeching halt, every time I saw him. All I wanted to do was continue exercising. I stopped each and every time he beckoned for me, not wanting to appear rude.

He would sit outside on the bench, by the water, smoking a cigarette and drinking his beer, while his small dog, or as he called him, *my wife's dog*, ran amuck around the pond. I was in constant fear that dog would eventually get eaten by an alligator.

We would have random light-hearted conversations about this or that and on a few occasions, he attempted to get philosophical. But, it was hard to take him seriously due to his slurred speech and red eyes. I suffered through it for the sake of being neighborly.

This one particular day, though, he flagged me down with a hand gesture and told me that I looked like I ate a lot of bread, from the looks of my backside. His comment was tactless. (I'm completely watering it down, not to offend anyone reading this.)

His statement took me aback. I stood there for a moment, assessing the situation. I was unsure whether I should feel offended by his crass evaluation of my derriere or if I should laugh it off and chalk it up to the fact that my neighbor was drunk, once again.

He went on to explain his logic. I listened to him decipher between the meat eaters and the bread eaters and I must admit, I became intrigued by his theory.

By the end of that conversation, I decided to considerably cut back on the dough products and like magic, the weight began to automatically fall off. I could not believe how much weight I had lost, so quickly. After inadvertently realizing that bread was one of the main culprits in my diet, I was able to significantly cut back enough to reach my goal weight.

1. *Eating for your digestion*

All good health starts with digestion

Poor digestion contributes to vitamin and mineral deficiencies, making it difficult for your body to fully absorb nutrients, which can inhibit weight loss. Your digestion works best when the sun is at its strongest peak, between 10am and 2pm. Lunch should be your largest meal and eaten by 2pm. Dinner should be eaten by 7pm.

Tips for better digestive health:

- Eat a diet rich in whole foods (fruits, vegetables, whole grains)
- Eat raw beets to thin your bile
- Choose lean meats
- Limit foods high in fat
- Hydrate (pure filtered or spring water) Drink one cup of water one half hour before each meal and one cup of water two hours after each meal.
- Drink warm or room temperature water, never ice-cold water
- Eat a high-fiber diet (insoluble and soluble)
- Don't smoke
- Avoid excessive caffeine and alcoholic beverages
- Eat probiotic foods (raw, unfiltered apple cider vinegar, buttermilk, yogurt, miso, tempeh, unpasteurized cheese)
- Eat fermented foods (sauerkraut, kefir, kombucha, kimchi)
- Eat on a schedule (same time every day)
- Minimize raw foods

- Leave one-third to one-quarter of your stomach empty

2. Get inflammation under control

There is a link between inflammation and obesity. When your immune system goes out of balance, you become susceptible to inflammation that can wreak havoc, causing chronic fire inside your body, which contributes to weight gain.

Ways to decrease inflammation:

- Reduce sugar intake
- Reduce stress
- Exercise
- Switch from unhealthy oils and fats to healthy oils and fats
- Trade in refined grains for whole grains
- Address your gut
- Avoid food allergens
- Eat dark leafy greens daily
- Eat fatty fish, nuts, berries, beets, ginger, turmeric, garlic, onions, olive oil, and tart cherries

3. Low Fat v's Low Carb Diet

If you have the obesity gene, you will be 2 ½ times more likely to become obese and it will be harder to lose weight than a person without this gene. In this case, following a low-fat diet is best to help you lose weight.

If you have diabetes, a low-carb diet is best to help you reach your weight loss goals.

4. Ways to manage your weight

a. Increase the efficiency of metabolism

Increase the quantity of nutrients in your diet to decrease appetite and increase metabolism. Increasing the efficiency of your metabolism happens naturally when we eat high-quality, unprocessed, real foods in their natural state, like fruits, vegetables, nuts, seeds, sprouts, sea vegetables, wheat grass, herbs and superfoods; all raw and organic, if possible.

b. Portion control

One of the major factors that can help you achieve your weight loss goals is proper portion control. Practicing portion control can help you feel satisfied eating less food. Eating smaller portions but eating more often will help glucose and insulin levels stabilize. Eating smaller portions can curb cravings and help reduce overall caloric intake.

Ways to control your portions:

- Eat salad to avoid overeating
- Split up trigger foods and leftovers into single serving portions
- Make your meat the side dish instead of main dish
- Serve yourself up to 20% less food than normal
- Order kids sized meal when you eat out
- Eat on a salad plate instead of a full sized plate
- Never eat snack food out of the box or bag it came in

c. Monitor your weight

Self-monitoring is critical for success when attempting to lose weight.

- One of the most effective ways to maintain your weight is to weigh yourself twice a week, using a scale (some people find this counterproductive and can feel discouraged if they haven't lost any weight) Use this method, only if you can handle the truth.
- Eat foods that are high in fiber (whole grain cereals, legumes, vegetables and fruits)
- Keep a food diary, exercise logs and pedometer

d. Get some ZZ's

Sleep and metabolism are controlled by the same sectors of the brain. On average, the less you sleep, the more you weigh. Insufficient sleep impacts your hunger hormones, causing an increase in appetite.

e. Drink White Tea

White tea has countless health benefits, but is best known for weight loss, by increasing metabolism and encouraging the body to burn more fat. It contains powerful antioxidants that prevent new fat cells from forming and fights signs of aging, like wrinkles.

5. Enjoy the process

How you eat is just as important as what you eat

In Japan, the Japanese perfected the art of the tea ceremony. The essence of this privileged ceremony has made it a tender reflection on life. The fundamentals of the ceremony lies in the humility of the guests, appreciating every single moment, in terms of time, place, season and those present and the art of simplicity and balance in form, movement and objects. In the tea ceremony, humility and respect are expected of the guests and the host. The door to the tea house is a low crawl space that requires all who enter to bow and humble themselves before entering the precious space. The unique nature of each tea ceremony is something to be cherished. The ceremony is special because although a person may take part in many ceremonies over his or her lifetime, there will never be a chance to recreate the same experience, with the same group of people, using the same settings and utensils, during the same time of day in the same season or even at the very unique time of their own life and experience. Every detail is to be savored because it cannot ever be the same with regards to simplicity and balance. Every aspect of the tea ceremony supports these ideals. Nothing in the tea room is unnecessary, loud or garish, in order to not distract from the present moment. Simple colors and design in clothing, artwork on the walls and floral arrangements are all ideal. Every moment of the tea ceremony, whether performed by the host or the guests is perfected to be the most simple and minimal act possible.

This Japanese tea tradition details every facet of appreciation one could have for being present and for living in the moment. Learn to appreciate your eating experience.

Ways to bring appreciation to your eating experience:

a. Appreciate your food

Before you eat, allow yourself a moment of thanks for your food and truly feel grateful to have a meal sitting there in front of you, when there are many hungry, less-fortunate people in the world. Use all of your senses and allow yourself to be stimulated. Look at your meal endearingly, admire the ingredients, savor the smell and enjoy the pleasant aroma. Taste it and feel the textures in your mouth, hear the crunch. Truly enjoy every morsel on your plate.

b. Eat at a moderate pace
(being within reasonable limits; not excessive or extreme; not too fast nor too slow)

It takes about 20 minutes from the time you begin eating for your brain to send out signals of fullness. Eating slowly, allows sufficient time to activate the signal from your brain and when you feel full, you eat less. Decelerating your bite rate improves your fat loss hormones, aiding digestion. When you take your time, you are able to easily remember what you ate, and how it tasted, forming a pleasurable eating experience in your mind.

c. Eat in a settled environment

Eating should be a sacred experience. Sit down, relax and bring awareness to yourself and to your food. Find a quiet place. Avoid too much conversation, watching television, sitting on the computer, loud music, and even reading at this time. This should be a time to observe, enjoy and appreciate each bite of food that you eat.

d. Never eat when you are upset

First things first, take a few slow, deep, even breaths to put your entire brain into a state of calm. Remember, the brain and gut are intimately connected and goes both ways. The gastrointestinal track is sensitive to emotion. Anger, anxiety, sadness, fear and other reckless emotions can trigger unwanted symptoms in the gut. And, when your gut is unhealthy it can send signals to the brain, causing stress, anxiety or depression.

e. Eat only when you feel hungry

How do you know if you're hungry?

- Ask yourself this question: Do you long for any food right now or just that very tempting food? If you would be satisfied to eat any food, then you could be hungry, instead of falling victim to your cravings.
- Don't mistake hunger for thirst. Drink a cup of water and then re-evaluate your hunger.
- Eat only after your previous meal has been digested. If you just ate your last meal less than two hours ago, chances are, you are not hungry.
- Allot yourself 10 minutes before eating when you feel hungry to see if the desire to eat has passed. You may just be experiencing a craving.

f. Eat until satisfied, not full

Eating until you are satisfied, not full, not only has weight loss benefits but digestion benefits, too. Eating until satisfied helps you save room for water and the expansion of gas for digestion.

- Leave one-third to one-quarter of your stomach empty.
- Pause halfway through your meal to gage your hunger level.
- Ask yourself throughout your meal, "Am I still hungry?"

g. Eat at the same time every day

When you don't eat at the same time every day, your body gets confused, not knowing where it's next meal will come from. The body then goes into stress mode, causing the stress hormone cortisol to be secreted. High levels of cortisol can lead to spikes in insulin, which causes inflammation and can increase your risk of cancer.

h. Always sit down to eat

Sitting when you eat allows you a chance to slow down and become aware of yourself and the food you are about to put into your body.

Weight Loss Juice Recipe

Apple
2 cups of spinach
Cucumber
2 leafs of (red) Cabbage
¼ pineapple
½ Lemon

4.

Stress Management

▼

Transform your thinking, transform your behavior;
transform your life

Stress is the number one epidemic in our civilization. Stress management is about changing your behavior, so that you can reduce bad stress. It involves avoiding stressful situations when you can and adjusting your reaction when you can't. Stress management can teach you healthy ways to deal with stress, help you reduce its dangerous effects, and inhibit stress from spiraling out of control.

1. What is stress?

First things first, let's clarify the myth that all stress is a bad thing. It's not. Stress is a natural human response designed to help us. When your body feels stressed, it thinks it's under attack and shifts to 'fight or flight' mode. It then releases certain hormones and chemicals such as adrenaline, cortisol and norepinephrine to prepare the body for physical action. This causes a number of reactions, from blood being diverted to muscles to shutting down bodily functions that are not immediately essential, such as digestion and your immune system. There are also biological effects; your blood pressure goes up, you get arrhythmia, your immune system is compromised, and your heart rate speeds up.

2. Good stress v's Bad stress

You might not be able to remove all the stressful things from your life, but you can change how you respond to them.

Stress isn't all bad. It can be described as a burst of energy that advises you on what to do when you find yourself in a situation, from something so simple as taking an exam or something more urgent, like running from a lion, tiger or bear.

In small doses, stress can have many advantages; such as motivating you to reach your goals and helping you achieve tasks more proficiently. Some stress can even strengthen the immune system. But, too much stress can be detrimental. Stress affects everyone differently.

There are two main types of stress:

- Good stress is meant to be motivating and beneficial
- Bad stress causes anxiety and other health problems

3. Nine common health problems caused by bad stress

a. Anxiety
b. Depression
c. Gastrointestinal problems (chronic heartburn- gastroesophageal reflux disease-irritable bowel syndrome)
d. High blood pressure
e. Headaches

f. Obesity
g. Heart attacks
h. The aging process
i. Premature death

4. *Causes of stress*

- Mistreatment
- Annoyances
- Conflict
- Overworked-Underappreciated
- Mortgage
- Wrong career
- Debt
- Deadlines
- Anxiety
- Taxes
- Poor leadership
- Expectations
- Relationship troubles
- Business predicaments

a. The Sympathetic Nervous System (fight or flight)

This system activates the adrenal medulla, which releases hormones into the bloodstream causing the body to speed up and become tense, as well as more alert. This system prepares you to fight, by providing you with more glycogen, which is converted to glucose. Your heartrate increases, pupils dilate, muscles contract and saliva production is reduced. Your bronchial tubes in your lungs dilate and digestive enzymes are inhibited. When the body is in fight or flight mode, its self-repairing mechanisms get shut off and your body can't heal itself.

b. Parasympathetic Nervous System (relaxation)

This system restores the body to a state of calmness and allows it to relax and repair itself. The parasympathetic nervous system controls the 'rest and digest' functions of the body.

5. Ways to decrease stress in your life

A tranquil heart is life to the body.

Stress is an inevitable part of life. It's impossible to eliminate, but learning to manage it is key.

a. Get out of debt

Having bill collectors call you all times of the day and night is not only draining but stressful, especially if you don't have the money to pay them.

b. Don't take on too much

Sometimes you just have to say, NO! You can't please everyone, all the time.

c. Trade in perfection for progress

Don't focus on the negative aspects, like everything that could go wrong, but instead, place your attention on moving forward, one healthy achievement at a time.

d. Resist the urge to think, *what if*

Stop playing out scenarios in your head that have not happened yet and probably won't. You will inadvertently make yourself more anxious by conjuring up fictitious situations with negative consequences. Instead, try this psychotherapy method, where you change your prospective about your particular fear. When you feel panic about a future situation, imagine in advance, how you want it to turn out. Envision it in full detail, even the outcome. Then, let go and let God.

e. Organize your life

Start with a room in your home that you've been meaning to organize, like your closet. Then, move on to another. Too much clutter can cause stress. You can't find anything because of your hoarding, and life becomes a hassle. Throw away old, broken items, donate clothes you haven't worn in a year or have a garage sale.

6. *Ways to manage stress*

a. Build up your stress defense shield

Disconnect your immune system from the stress of this world by way of nutrition; eating whole living foods and superfoods.

- Raw Cacao
- Mucuna
- Maca
- Blue Green Algae
- Chlorella
- Spirulina

- Bee Pollen
- Royal Jelly
- Hemp Seeds
- Goji Berries
- Medicinal Mushrooms
- Marine Phytoplankton

b. Address nutritional deficiencies

Being under a lot of stress can deplete your vitamins and minerals. Taking the time to figure out which nutrients you are deficient in can reduce and/or eliminate stress, anxiety and depression.

Dark chocolate (soluble fiber & minerals), bananas (amino acid tryptophan which is converted into serotonin), blueberries & blackberries (vitamin C), Strawberries (magnesium), salmon (omega-3 fatty acid), kiwi (vitamin C), whole grains (vitamin B), oatmeal (complex carbohydrates boost serotonin levels), oranges (vitamin C), avocado (potassium), green vegetables (calcium), almonds (vitamins B & E) and milk (vitamin D).

c. Get enough sleep

Obey your circadian rhythm which is your internal body clock. Around 9 pm every night, your brain secretes a hormone called melatonin which is produced by the pineal gland or third eye. Artificial lighting from televisions, computer screens, and cellphones can disrupt the production of melatonin, making it hard to fall asleep. The production of melatonin is needed to signal to your body that it's time to wind down for the night, getting you ready for sleep.

It is imperative to **decalcify your pineal gland** by eliminating sodium fluoride from your diet. This chemical is prevalent in our food, drinking water, bath water, toothpaste, mouthwash, excess sugar and sweeteners and even regular exposure to cell phones. Fluoride builds up in your body over time and causes a decrease in melatonin production which can then cause sleep deprivation disorders, like insomnia.

One way to get more sleep is to **eliminate caffeine** from your diet. Too much caffeine can cause headaches, sleep deprivation and anxiety.

The vicious cycle of anxiety causing symptoms that cause further anxiety that cause further symptoms is part of why this disorder is so hard to overcome or control. If you're a coffee or tea drinker, switch to decaf.

Create a bedtime ritual and stick to a schedule. Don't eat or drink within two hours of bedtime. Turn your bedroom into a Feng Shui, sleep-inducing environment. Take the TV out of the bedroom and only use the room for intimacy and sleep. Keep your room dark, quiet and cool. Clear your head of negative thoughts; postpone worrying and brainstorming. Practice relaxation techniques, like deep breathing and muscle relaxation before bedtime. Improve your sleep environment; making sure your mattress and pillows are comfortable and provide you with proper neck and back support.

d. Exercise regularly

Regular exercise will independently lower your risk for many health problems. People who exercise have better moods and more energy than people who don't. Practically, any form of exercise will increase your fitness level while decreasing your stress.

When choosing an exercise routine, it's helpful to select one that you truly enjoy—whether it's swimming, playing tennis, jogging, some form of martial arts or just brisk walking. To delight in what you do makes it easier to stick with it long-term.

For a new level of motivation and commitment, find a friend to partner with. From a fitness trainer at the gym, to your neighbor, maybe a coworker—exercising with someone is a powerful incentive to get out there and make it happen.

e. Do relaxation techniques

Stimulate your smell receptors by taking a warm aromatherapy bath. Use Epsom Salt and one or two of these essential oils (chamomile, benzoin, bergamot, cedarwood, clary sage, frankincense, geranium, jasmine, lavender, neroli, patchouli, rose, sandalwood and ylang ylang. Your emotions will become regulated as your body soaks for up to 40 minutes. (The first 20 minutes of soaking in Epsom Salt, releases toxins. The last 20 minutes, you will absorb magnesium).

Sit by a body of water while listening to meditation music. Listening and playing music increases the body's production of the antibody immunoglobulin A – the cells that attack viruses and help to boost the effectiveness of the immune system, as well as lowering cortisol. The object is to relax. De-stressing music like Reiki, Zen or Ayervedic meditation music works best. When I'm anxious or worried and choose to use music as my medicine, my favorite choice is classical. Listening to nature sounds is highly relaxing as well. It calms the nervous system.

Get a relaxation massage with sesame or almond oil. This is a century old Ayervedic tradition by cultures known for their longevity. Self-massage with this oil will strengthen your ability to handle stress by supporting the nervous system.

Massage the CV 17 Acupressure point (also known as 'the sea of tranquility' in Chinese medicine) to reduce stress and anxiety. It's located four finger widths north of the base of the breastbone, almost directly in the center of the chest.

Drink green, black or oolong tea which contains the amino acid, L- Theanine, a component that provides a calming effect by toning down some of the stimulating neurotransmitters that make you anxious.

f. Take some *ME* time

Reduce TV time to make time for prayer and meditation. Taking time to be one with your creator is essential for true happiness.

Take a 5-15 minute rest every day! When you quiet your mind, and detach from your emotions for just a few moments, you can experience renewed energy, improved mental clarity, enhanced creativity and more inner peace.

Do a good deed every day! Find someone to do something nice for and don't expect anything in return. Carry an elderly persons groceries to their car or let someone go ahead of you in line. Open your heart to this idea and watch the generosity flow. While others will appreciate your kind gestures, this exercise is really for you.

Get a pet! If you can afford to own a pet, get one and pet them often. They help normalize brain chemistry. From just a few minutes of stroking your pet prompts the release of a number of *feel good* hormones in humans, including serotonin, prolactin, dopamine and oxytocin; these hormones can slow heart rate and breathing, quiet blood pressure and inhibit the production of stress hormones.

Drive less! You can avoid all of the stressful situations related to driving. It doesn't just save on gas and auto repairs, but it has health benefits to help you stress less; like breathing in less pollution, avoiding accidents, eliminating road rage, no sitting in traffic or listening to loud horns honking, taking detours or getting a flat tire.

Find your life's purpose! Cultivate your spirituality. Think about your proudest achievements, what brings you joy and what you value most in life. By affirming your purpose and uncovering what's most meaningful in your life, you will begin to connect to your true passions and be able to discover what fulfills you.

Plant a garden! As you sow seeds to one day reap a harvest, you are also unavoidably nature bathing, which will expose you to sunlight while you breathe in fresh oxygenated air. Listen to the birds sing and the rustling of the trees blowing in the wind while directly connecting to God's green earth. Not to mention, the organic tasty fruits and vegetables you get to enjoy and the sense of accomplishment of knowing you created something great to sustain your health. If you can't go outside, open a window and look outside. If you aren't near a window, close your eyes and imagine it.

g. Practice Earthing

Earthing or grounding is a simple practice that neutralizes the positively charged electrons in our bodies by providing us with negative electrons which protects us from chronic inflammation and pain. The earth is the #1 antioxidant in the world with many health benefits, including improving auto-immune diseases. All you do is, sit, lay or stand barefoot on the earth's dirt, sand or grass. The longer you do it, the better the results. This is something you can do in your front or backyard, everyday all by yourself. Enjoy!

h. Breathe deeply

Deep breathing exercises are a great way to quickly lower cortisol levels. Grounding yourself helps create nervous system balance, and lessens stress, by inducing parasympathetic nervous system activity or relaxation response.

i. Visualization

Use a vision board to project what you want to attract into your life or just close your eyes and envision all the colorful details in your mind. If you want a new home, see yourself making delicious meals in the kitchen and allow yourself to actually smell the aroma. Hear the sounds of the birds chirping outside your kitchen window as you cut the vegetables and stir the pots. Feel your muscles relax as you dream this wonderful dream. Smile and believe it as if it is already so. Use all of your senses when using this visualization technique for faster manifestation. When you are finished visualizing, say *thank you* to your creator.

j. Get a job you love

Work related stress is at an all-time high these days and is responsible for over 50% of your stress. Think about it! You spend at least eight hours there, not to mention your commute to and from. Notice how your body feels; tense, agitated or anxious. Maybe you have unexplained aches and pains. Pay attention to any triggers you experience. Once you've figured out who or what is causing your stress, it's critical to address it and ultimately eliminate it; even if that means stepping down from a management position, changing departments or quitting altogether.

Take a moment, if possible to reevaluate your job situation and if it's feasible to start a new career doing something you love, go for it! You will know when you have the right job because it will never feel like work.

k. Accept the sweetness and the sorrow

Think of life as a test! When you go through challenges in life, think from a prospective of it just being a test that you intend to pass with flying colors.

l. Practice patience

There are three facets to patience:

- Persistence to keep going, even though you don't yet see the end result.
- Acceptance is being able to accept the fact that whatever is going on right now is the way it is.
- Peace or a state of calm in the face of what is.

m. Be slow to anger

Don't sweat the small stuff! When you get angry, your immune system is weakened, you have worse lung capacity and you're at three times the risk of having a stroke. And, if that's not bad enough, after an angry outburst, you double your risk for having a heart attack.

Think before you speak. Don't blurt out the first thing that comes to mind, not having thought through how you will come across to the other person. When you are angry, your filters become inhibited and the words that come from anger can cut like knife.

Take a time-out to yourself and regroup. If you feel yourself getting angry, go somewhere quiet where you can be alone and breathe. My favorite place to retreat is the bathroom, where I can acceptably lock the door for privacy. In there, I redirect my focus from what made me mad to how to find a possible solution.

n. Change your relationship with stress

The first step is to acknowledge your stress. Secondly, do not allow your mind to draw conclusions for you that probably won't even happen. Stay in the moment. Thirdly, change your belief about stress and how it will damage your health. Remember, what you believe is what you will receive. Lastly, continue to have high standards for excellence, but be sure to trade in perfection for progress.

o. Be present

Focus on the present. Stop worrying about the past. Be more conscious of life as it happens. Cherish all parts of your journey. Take your time; don't rush. Live slowly and savor each moment.

p. Let go of what you can't control

Control is rooted in fear. When you surrender, or let go and let God, you eliminate fear and stress from that moment. The more moments you allow this to happen, the more moments you will have in a state of peace and calm. Stop trying to make things happen and just let them happen.

q. Reframe the situation

Reframing means simply to change your prospective on a given situation, by replacing a negative thought with a positive one in order to put yourself in a positive and resourceful state of mind. You cannot always change the things that happen to you in life, but making the decision to change the way you view those situations are crucial.

Ways to positively reframe a situation:

- Ask yourself, "What is this situation trying to teach me?"
- Know that, problems are just challenges
- Face your fears head on (or that negative emotion)

r. Be grateful

Gratitude means thankfulness; noticing the simple pleasures around you, counting your blessings and acknowledging everything that you receive. Practicing gratitude is a soothing way to experience life. It's a means to connect with life by allowing yourself to feel grateful at the present moment.

s. Journal

Journaling is a way to get things off your chest. Taking a few moments to stop and be grateful for all of the positive things in your life will give you an immediate sense of relief from stress. There's always something you can be grateful for, like your health, your family and friends, your food, your home and your job. Even if you're in poor health, with no friends or family, you're homeless without a job and nothing to eat, you can still be grateful you are alive and are able to see the sun which brightens up the world and showers you with vitamin D; music to lift your spirits when you feel down; oxygen so you can breathe; nature for making our world a beautiful place to live in. Being grateful even for the pain you have suffered which has made you stronger person. You get the idea.

t. Share your feelings

In addition to journaling, recent research indicates that talking to someone with similar circumstances as you, can greatly reduce stress, by allowing you to vent to someone whom understands what you're going through.

7. How I manage stress in my life

My husband and I come from two very different cultures. I'm a southern belle and he's a fast-paced east coaster. When we married, most of our quarrels were communication conflicts. He saw the world one way, and I perceived it a completely different way, which caused wear and tear on our marriage. When arguments ensued, I spent my day feeling anxious and heartbroken. My husband is the type to say what he has to say and be done with it. Me, on the other hand, I can literally brood for days at a time; going back and forth in my head, playing back the conversation, over and over again. Meanwhile, he's in the living room belly laughing at a television show.

We are both sensitive people and we sometimes tend to hurt each other's feelings, even though it's not our intention. Once we realized that, we changed how we responded to one another and also thought before we reacted. I know he didn't say those things to hurt me, It just didn't feel good to me, for whatever reason and vice versa.

One day, I decided to stop reacting and respond with compassion. I noticed, when I responded to him negatively, it made him defensive. When I responded with compassion, he kept calm and we were able to continue having a normal conversation without anyone snapping on the other. Before I knew it, Michael followed suit and life together is better than ever. We are still a work in progress, but we implement the same tips given in this book and it has made our relationship so much healthier.

Sleep Inducing Juice Recipe

1 large orange, unpeeled
½ bunch watercress
7 celery stalks
½ head romaine lettuce
5 almonds
5 whole walnuts

5.

Smoking Cessation

▼

Every time you say NO to a cigarette, you're saying,
YES to life

1. Who should read this chapter?

You may think, if you are not a smoker, you should skip this whole chapter. *NO! Please don't...*

This chapter has two main benefits:

- We all know someone who smokes and wants to quit; whether a friend, family member, neighbor or coworker. This chapter could save someone's life.
- A lot of the same tips given in this chapter can be used to replace smoking with alcoholism, drug use or any other addiction.

Smoking is a chronic condition that may require repeated interventions over many years. On average, smokers attempt to quit three or four times over seven to 10 years before they achieve long-term maintenance. That is because **smoking is an addiction**.

Part of the reason why nicotine is so addictive is, it permeates your system as a toxin and becomes extremely hard to remove.

The brain gets hooked on nicotine, and when you use it, it causes blood vessels to constrict in your body. Applying natural ways to dilate blood vessels and improve your circulation, is key!

Seek the help of an experienced herbalist to prescribe the proper herbs and dosages that will dilate your blood vessels.

14 natural ways to dilate blood vessels:

- Quit smoking
- Control blood pressure naturally
- Control cholesterol
- Control diabetes
- Maintain good dental hygiene
- Hyperbaric Oxygen Therapy
- Stretching
- Exercise
- Sweat in an infrared sauna
- Use essential oil of lemon
- Eat temperature hot food
- Eat curcumin
- Consume low dosages of alcoholic beverages
- Follow an anti-inflammatory diet, such as the *Modern Paleo Diet.*

Five ways to improve blood circulation:

- Eat ginger, garlic and onion
- Eat foods rich in magnesium
- Fresh rosemary
- Perfect your posture

- Reduce stimulants (coffee, tea, energy drinks, cigarettes, diet pills)

Although nicotine dependence is the primary reason people have trouble quitting, here are seven other factors that play a role in unsuccessful cessation:

- Genetics
- Habitual behavior
- Socioeconomic factors
- High anxiety and stress levels
- Spouse smokes
- Being addicted to *menthol* cigarettes (which are harder to quit)
- Insatiable cravings

Cravings can be strong and people often relapse because they don't know how to curb their urges. One way to combat cravings is to replace nicotine with all natural foods and herbal supplements that do the exact same thing.

Don't be discouraged if you make multiple attempts to quit and relapse. This happens often and to many people. The key is to figure out what caused the setback; your emotions, the setting you were in or a fight with your spouse. Once you can identify the trigger, the key is to try to avoid that trigger the next time. Keep trying again and again, over and over, until you are successful. Do not give up. Set another quit date within the month and try again. Believe that it will happen for you. Be patient with yourself.

Some of the smoking cessation techniques listed here may feel unrealistic to you, but they have been proven to work. As you scroll further down the list, take notes of the methods you feel are feasible for you to try. Take your time and be strategic. Do what feels good to your spirit. If you don't feel good about having to limit your time from certain friends, then don't do it. Try one of the other simple behavioral modification strategies, instead. Keep in mind, the first three days are the most difficult, so you may have to put forth more effort, during this time.

If you prepare your mind and realize, quitting smoking will probably be one of the most difficult tasks of your entire life, you'll be more apt to tackle more of the challenges with ease.

2. Five successive stages to quitting

Smokers generally go through five stages when trying to quit smoking; each involving different challenges and issues. Identify your current step and then try to advance yourself to the next step.

Pre-contemplation stage (not thinking about quitting)
Contemplation stage (thinking about quitting, but not quite ready)
Preparation stage (getting ready to quit)
Active stage (actively taking steps to quit)
Maintenance (remaining a non-smoker)

3. What happens to your body when you quit smoking

- **In 20 minutes**, your heart rate and blood pressure will stabilize

- In **8-12 hours**, your blood oxygen levels will return to normal
- In **24 hours,** your risk for coronary artery disease will reduce.
- In **48 hours**, you decrease your risk of heart attack. Your nerve ending will begin to grow, regenerating your senses of smell and taste.
- In **72 hours**, your energy levels increase and bronchial tubes relax and all nicotine will be completely out of your body.
- In **2 weeks**, your circulation increases and continues to improve for 10 weeks
- In **1 month,** the cilia inside your lungs will begin to repair.
- In **3-9 months**, your brain chemistry returns to normal and your lung capacity improves by 10%, causing coughing, wheezing and breathing issues to dissipate.
- In **1 year**, your risk for having a heart attack will drop by half.
- In **5 years**, your risk of having a stroke returns to that of a non-smoker.
- In **10 years**, your risk of lung cancer will return to that of a non-smoker.
- In **15 years**, your risk of having a heart attack and pancreatic cancer will return to that of a non-smoker.
- In **20 years,** female risk of death from all smoking related causes including lung disease and cancer is now that of a non-smoker.

This timeline applies to everyone, as long as you stop the self-destruction in time.

4. How I quit smoking

I was a smoker, so I know first-hand how challenging it can be to quit. I tried for many years and on countless occasions to put my addiction behind me by using the patch, chewing the gum, going cold turkey or weaning myself off of them slowly. Over the years, I have tossed many packs of smokes into the trash. I even tried fasting from cigarettes for three days at a time, but to no avail. I would constantly revert back to my old ways for one reason or another.

I recall quitting for several weeks to months at a time, and during those times, my sense of smell improved. I was then able to smell the unpleasant smoky odor on other people after they had smoked, when they entered the elevator or whizzed past me. I honestly remember thinking, "Oh God, did I smell like that?" While in transition, during an off smoking period, I reveled in knowing how good I smelled and it became an incentive for me to stay clean.

Cigarette smoke gives off an awful smell. It gets into everything, from your hair, to your clothes, to your furniture, especially if you smoke in the house; not to mention the poor little pets that live with in-house smokers.

I smoked in my car and then went to work every day, I'm certain, smelling like a puff of smoke. The horror my clients must've endured.

I recall, one day, I arrived at work and a family of five came in and handed over a little boy to me who needed a haircut. He looked to be about eight years old. His mother, grandmother and siblings left him in my care while they waited in the car.

The smell was unbelievable. He reeked of cigarette smoke that had attached itself to his hair, clothes and body. It smelled as though, he, himself was a smoker.

I rushed him to the shampoo bowl and scrubbed vigorously, to remove as much of the stench from his hair, as possible. I didn't know what else to do. I felt so sad for him.

When I finished his haircut, his mother stepped in to pay. I watched them drive off into the sunset. His mother and grandmother both puffed on their cigarettes and all of the windows to the minivan were rolled up tightly.

I was concerned for him, wondering if he would get to grow up or if his life would be cut short from second hand smoke at the hands of his own mother and grandmother. I grew angry at them for their selfish behavior, exposing the children to those toxic poisons in a car where that is all their lungs would breathe in. That little boy and his unfortunate situation, lingered in my mind, for a long time after meeting them.

There were so many reasons why I wanted to quit smoking; I knew it wasn't good for me, I smelled badly, I did not want to disappoint my parents, I wanted to be a better role model for my son, I wanted to please God, I wanted to save the money I spent on cigarettes, and so on.

I was able to quit for a while, but then I relapsed because I hadn't made any real lifestyle changes, which is a key component for quitting, for good.

My original mindset was to use nicotine replacement therapy, which helped to physically lessen my nicotine intake, but I felt guilty because I knew that all of those over-the-counter cessation products were full of unnatural chemicals that filled my body with even more toxins. So, I decided to try natural strategies and I'm happy to report, it finally stuck.

5. How to take action against those cigarettes

a. Find your reason

In order to get motivated to quit for good this time, you need a powerful reason. Choose a reason that is stronger than your urge to smoke like the health and welfare of your children or grandkids or even how much money you can save.

b. Avoid stress

Stress is unavoidable in our world today, but it is also one of the main reasons people find it so hard to quit smoking. You must avoid stress as best as you can. Ask your spouse to get on board with a no-argue policy for the first few weeks of you quitting. Find ways to unwind and exercises that help you blow off steam. Only talk to those friends who make you laugh and feel good, not the ones carrying around all of life's problems and are full of negative energy.

c. Eat more organic fruits and vegetables

Add more fruits and vegetables to your plate to help load your body with essential vitamins and nutrients you need that have been depleted from smoking. Do not diet during smoking cessation because you don't want to deprive yourself of too many things at once. This could have an unfavorable effect, causing it to backfire.

d. Take vitamin C

Smoking only one cigarette uses up approximately 25 mg of vitamin C, which can help flush toxic heavy metals as well as nicotine from the body. This vitamin will provide your body a lot of support during smoking cessation and help restore function to blood vessels which have been damaged by years of smoking. You should supplement with this vitamin as you prepare to quit and continue taking it for a few months after you have successfully quit. Citrus fruits are a great source of vitamin C, which has been depleted from your body due to smoking. It can also cut cigarette cravings.

e. Take magnesium

Smoking causes stress, which in turn causes cholesterol levels to rise and magnesium levels to drop. Taking magnesium will relieve stress and anxiety.

f. Avoid sugar

Many smokers feel a strong urge for sweet foods after quitting smoking because sweets can help curb cravings. If this is the case for you, choose low calorie treats, like fruit, sugar-free gelatin, plain yogurt sweetened with berries or a scoop of sorbet.

g. Do mindfulness meditation

This meditation technique encourages you to live a healthy lifestyle and people who do it are able to normalize their cravings, have less withdrawal symptoms or stress and are able to get their emotions under control.

h. Take vitamin E

Vitamin E protects tissues and cell membranes and repairs cell damage caused by cigarette smoking. This vitamin neutralizes cancer-promoting free radicals in the lungs.

i. Take B vitamin complex

Smoking depletes the body of B vitamins. They help to normalize and calm your nervous system. In addition, it can relieve stress and fatigue. B vitamins can have a favorable effect on anxiety and insomnia that is usually associated with smoking cessation.

j. Reduce caffeine consumption

When quitting smoking, reduce your caffeine intake or if possible, eliminate it altogether. Switch to decaf coffee and tea. Nicotine reduces the effects of caffeine in the body, which means, when you quit smoking, the same amount of caffeine can have more than a 50% stronger effect on you. Over consumption of caffeine can worsen anxiety and other withdrawal symptoms.

k. Use cayenne pepper (or black)

Cayenne is a sulfur product and will remove tar resin from your lungs by detoxifying the carbon left over in your lungs from smoking tobacco. You can eat it with food or mix it with water and drink it.

l. Hypnosis

During hypnosis for smoking cessation, a patient is often asked to imagine unpleasant outcomes from smoking. They can also be taught self-hypnosis and then asked to repeat certain affirmations when the desire to smoke arises.

m. Exercise

Exercise limits weight gain by decreasing your appetite and helping you cope with cravings. Even moderate activity can ease withdrawal symptoms, especially, within the first three days to about a week. Plus, it helps to overcome the psychological hooks.

n. Try acupuncture

There is a powerful acupuncture point located on the inside of the arm, above the wrist, called Tim Mee that is used specifically to help a patient stop smoking, by altering the taste of the cigarette. But, it must be used alongside other points for perfect balance.

o. Self-massage

You can reduce your cravings for smoking by doing a two minute self-massage on your hands and/or ears. When giving yourself an ear massage, it will release endorphins, which are natural painkillers.

p. Take herbal supplements

Various herbs can dilate artery walls and decrease blood pressure. Licorice root is an excellent choice to satisfy oral cravings. *Contact a professional herbalist to get an herbal therapy session for smoking cessation.*

q. Identify your triggers

Daily life can be filled with triggers, especially if you are a long time smoker. For the first weeks of quitting, you must identify those situations that cause you to reach for your smokes.

Common triggers are:

- Stress and the effect it has on your emotions
- Being in the company of other smokers in social settings
- Smoking at certain times of day
- Particular food or drink can be associated with smoking
- Happy hour after work on Fridays with coworkers
- Boredom
- Driving
- Walking the dog
- Watching TV

r. Change your habits

If you associate your morning coffee with a cigarette, switch to tea or juice. If you like to smoke after a meal, try taking a walk, instead. If you take smoke breaks at work, switch it up and grab a non-smoking coworker to chat with. If you like to smoke while on the phone with friends, don't call them until you are strong enough to resist your triggers.

s. Change your friends

Make sure to have a conversation with your friends to let them know, you aren't avoiding them, though you are avoiding situations that might make you want to smoke. Seek the company of your non-smoking friends when you are quitting, to avoid any temptations.

t. Stop buying cartons

It is an absolute true fact, that buying most things in bulk rewards you with a few extra dollars in your pocket, in the long run. However, you will smoke more cigarettes when you know you have more packs waiting for you in the freezer.

u. Switch brands

If you are a menthol smoker, there is nothing worse than running out of cigarettes and having to bum one from someone who smokes non-menthol and vice versa. The next time you run out, switch brands. You should be completely turned off toward cigarettes after that.

v. Give up alcohol

Drinking and smoking for many people go hand in hand. Until you are strong enough to resist the urge to smoke, you may have to give up your afternoon cocktails. Going to the club on

the weekends may have to come to an end, too. No wine tast-
ings on date night or going to the winery as a weekend getaway.
No mimosa's for Sunday brunch or Irish coffee after dinner. If
you cannot give up alcohol completely for the first few weeks
of quitting, try to limit it.

w. Drink plenty water

Water is a natural detoxifier and will speed up the detoxifying
process while helping you heal. Your body needs water to coun-
teract many of the harmful effects of nicotine and tobacco. De-
hydration is linked to increased cravings. Also, the toxins from
the nicotine causes you to have cravings. Once you've completely rid yourself of all traces of nicotine, the cravings and
withdrawal symptoms should cease.

x. Clean your house

Remove smoking paraphernalia! Get rid of any and everything
associated with smoking; cigarette packs, ash-trays, lighters
and cases. Throw old butts into the toilet, so you cannot go
later to retrieve them from the trashcan. Sweep and mop the
house to remove any smells that will prompt you to want to
smoke. Wash clothes that smell like smoke. Clean your carpets,
upholstery and draperies that hold smoke odors that you've become nose-blind to. Clean your car of smoke smells and replace
it with nice, fresh fragrances. Your goal is to remove that famil-
iar scent from your immediate life; your home, car, clothes, fur-
nishings, and even your pets, who could probably use a bath.
You don't want to see or smell anything that reminds you of
smoking.

y. Get support

People who feel supported are more likely to quit smoking for good. Ask for help from friends or family members that you trust will encourage you to keep going. Join a support group or seek behavioral therapy from a counselor. Make an appointment with me, or your local wellness coach that will help identify triggers and stick to smoking cessation strategies. If you do not have anyone that you can rely on for support, please hear me loud and clear...YOU CAN DO IT! I did it and yes, it was very hard. But, now that it's done, I do not regret quitting.

Vitamin C Juice Recipe

½ head of broccoli
1 cup of spinach
½ lemon
1 cucumber
8 strawberries

6.

Emotional Health

▼

Cultivate the Attitude of Gratitude

The thinking mind produces over 60,000 thoughts per day and 85% of them are the same thoughts we had yesterday.

Caring for your emotional health is just as important as caring for your physical health. Negative emotions are the root cause of many health problems that could have been prevented, if only you would have known exactly what to do. Luckily, it's not too late. You can convert your negative thoughts into positive ones. This will drastically change the outcome of your quality of life.

The average American has 50 or more stress responses a day. Your body is equipped with natural, self-repair mechanisms that repair broken proteins, kill cancer cells, fight infections, prevent aging, and maintain the homeostasis of the body.

1. *Nurturing your emotions*

- Spend time with people that make you feel good about yourself
- Do something nice for someone else
- Wear colors that you love and make you feel good
- Do things that showcase your special skills and talents

- Listen to your body and give it what it needs to feel good
- Eat healthy foods
- Exercise
- Forgive yourself
- Let go of negative emotions; guilt, fear and shame

2. Curing v's Healing

Curing is for the physical body and healing is for the mind.

- Curing is a renewal of health, symptoms are nonexistent, and a remedy of disease.
- Healing is not the removal of symptoms, but rather an integrative process that goes beyond the physical and includes mental, emotional, and spiritual wellness.

3. Heal your emotions

Your ideal goal is to be emotionally free. Free of all resentments and anger, guilt and shame.

a. Take time to laugh often

Not only does laughter burn calories, it decreases stress hormones, increases immune cells and infection-fighting antibodies which improves your resistance to disease by triggering the release of endorphins.

Laugh often! Strive for fifteen minutes of laugh time a day. Real hard belly laughs are even better. Watch comical movies and think back on memories that tickle your funny bone. Call friends on the phone who are witty and pleasant, not the ones who zap your energy with all of their personal problems.

b. Say heartfelt affirmations

Allowing your ears to hear what your mouth says is a great way to get control of your wandering emotions and to feel good instantly. Still, you must believe what you are saying for it to work. As you're saying positive affirmations, smile and feel your request as if it has already come to pass.

c. Have hope and faith

Having both hope and faith allows you to feel that something great is waiting for you at the end of the tunnel, helping you push through difficult times.

d. Forgiveness

Human behavior suggests that humans are wired to want revenge when they have been hurt by another person. When our pride or self-esteem gets injured, we want compensation for the damages.

There are numerous scriptures in the bible on forgiveness. Forgiving others releases us from anger and allows us to receive the healing we need. Forgiving those who hurt us is the key to personal peace of mind.

e. Be optimistic

Look on the bright side of things. This will help you to feel happy in your day-to-day life and help you better cope with stress.

f. Learn EFT (emotional freedom technique)

EFT is a form of acupressure, based on the same energy meridians used in traditional acupuncture to treat physical as well as emotional ailments, without using needles.

g. Accept yourself

Seek out and embrace the positive traits about yourself and avoid measuring your worth by comparing yourself to someone else.

h. Love your body

If your body feels that you love it, it will love you back by doing everything in its power to keep it alive and well. Point the lens at things that are great about yourself. Are you smart, funny or creative? Find things about yourself that are of value and appreciate them, as well as your weaknesses. These things as a whole make you who you are. You are unique. No two people are alike.

Find activities that you enjoy and can thrive in. Take your time and ask yourself questions to determine what they are. Do you enjoy indoor or outdoor activities? Are you creative? Do you like to work with your hands? Are you a white or blue collar individual? Do you enjoy activities that involve adventure? These are the types of questions to ask yourself when trying to discover what makes you happiest. Being happy is one of the best ways to love yourself.

Give yourself gifts! Whether it's treating yourself to a new outfit or spending more *me-time*. Listen to your body and give it what it needs to perform at its very best; like eating healthy foods, drinking enough water and getting enough rest.

7.

Operation Detox

▼

Eliminate more toxins from your body than you take in

Why I added The *Central Florida Operation Detox* Program to my wellness coaching repertoire

By the time you've reached this chapter, you will have read about the five main categories under the umbrella of wellness coaching; nutrition, fitness, weight management, stress management and smoking cessation. I chose to take it a step further and a little deeper.

My research has been very time consuming, yet worth every second I spent, uncovering hidden agendas of certain organizations. It is not my goal to name names or expose company secrets or their covert operations for adding poisonous chemicals to our air, water and food supply. However, I will offer you a plethora of tips on how to eliminate these toxins from your body that you are exposed to, without your consent. I urge you to take a deeper look at the carcinogens that are being put into our environment, deliberately, to cause sickness and disease, especially cancer.

Research is not a strong suit for everyone. So, I took the liberty of creating a program that allows me to go into the homes of my clients and make them aware of the toxins specific to their own home. It is a great privilege for me to share the information I've gathered with my clients, so they are well informed about the toxins that are lurking in their intimate surroundings. I detail ways to reduce and/or eliminate contaminants, by giving them alternate recommendations.

1. *How to eliminate more toxins from your body than you take in*

a. Eat plenty of fiber

Toxins tend to stick to the colon and intestines, which can have a negative effect on the body. A high-fiber diet helps to flush those toxins out, through elimination. If you get the daily recommended amount of fiber every day, especially from food, you can prevent some of the unnecessary toxic buildup.

- 25 grams (women)
- 38 grams (men)

b. Take herbal supplements

Seek an experienced herbalist to help you work toward reducing your toxicity levels.

c. Take vitamin C

Vitamin C is a critical weapon in the fight to release toxins from the bowels, and improve eliminations.

d. Reduce stress by emphasizing powerful emotions

For some people, the mind is a down-right dangerous place. Although, it doesn't have to be. When a problem rears its ugly head, spin it to find a solution. To change the way you think is essential to detox the brain.

Example: If you get stuck in traffic, instead of feeling frustrated, which will serve no good purpose, look at it as an opportunity for some unexpected prayer time.

e. Detoxify your lymphatic system

The lymphatic system is responsible for flushing out toxins and carrying waste away from the immune system. It is one of the most important, yet often forgotten, systems of the human body. The stronger the lymphatic system, the stronger and responsive your immune response and its defenses will be.

Because it does not have a pump to move, like blood, it has to rely on the muscles and joints being relaxed and contracted to move it. It can become stagnant when overwhelmed with toxins, which is why it is imperative to eliminate existing toxins as well as reduce future toxin intake by quitting smoking, not breathing in unclean air, drinking unfiltered water and by not eating chemically processed foods.

Ways to get your lymph flowing:

- **Get hydrated**
  Drink plenty of water to keep lymph moving; 8 cups of water a day. If you are dehydrated, (the leading cause of lymphatic system congestion), drink half your weight

in ounces of water a day. To take it a step further and expedite things, add lemon. More ways to encourage the movement of lymph is to:

- **Eat raw foods**
  Eating raw foods will help to quickly release toxins, especially if eaten on an empty stomach.
- **Sweat in a sauna**
  You release toxins when you sweat.
- **Get a lymphatic drainage massage**
  This type of massage physically helps the lymph to drain.
- **Practice yin yoga**
  Yin yoga requires you to hold poses from three to 10 minutes. You experience a change in gravity and differences in pressure to improve lymphatic flow.
- **Dry body brush yourself**
  Brush your largest organ, the skin, with a natural bristle brush to encourage the flow of lymph.
- **Breathe deeply**
  Take deep breaths from the lungs; in through the nose, out through the mouth. This allows oxygen to circulate more completely, throughout the body.
- **Walking**
  Just a simple walk can boost the flow of lymph. Breathe in as deeply as possible during your walk, to increase lymph flow.
- **Use a rebounder (mini trampoline)**
  The best way to get the lymphatic system moving is to exercise. Rebounding is the most effective form of exercise you can do. Jump on the rebounder between ten and twenty minutes every day.

- **Use an inversion table or chair**
  The health benefits of inversion therapy are many, ranging from physical, to mental. It boosts the immune system, improves digestion, the circulatory system and the respiratory system. It also has physical fitness and cosmetic benefits, too. To top it all off, it's another amazing way to progress the function of your lymphatic system. If you don't want to use inversion equipment, you can put your body in inversion positions to gain effective results. The yoga position, downward dog will invert the top half of your body and lying on your back on the floor with your feet on the wall will invert the bottom half of your body.

- **Take a hydrotherapy shower (use a shower filter)**
  This type of shower alternates the water temperature from hot to cold. Always start with hot and end with cold, while saturating your entire body. The hot water helps to relax you, while relieving stress and the cold water aids to relieve inflammation, and stimulates the removal of toxins from your skin and lymphatic system. Alternating the temperatures, moves the circulation in and out, unblocking stuck flows, increasing the rate of detoxification and moving nutrients to various parts of the body. Start by setting your water temperature at the hottest tolerable setting for five minutes and then turn it to the coldest tolerable setting for thirty seconds. Moving forward, each alternate temperature change should be for thirty seconds each. Repeat this process three to seven times.

- **Ladies, do not wear underwire bras**
  The wire in the bra will obstruct lymph flow and prevent normal drainage.

2. How I combat my toxins

Every birthday and Christmas my husband asks, "Babe, what do you want for your birthday?" I immediately answer, "An air purifier or shower filter or an electromagnetic field pendant." "What do you want for Christmas?" My reply was consistently along the same lines, "a non-stick cookware set or a glassware setup to replace all of our plastics containing BPA. All in fun, he asked, "What should I get you next year, a wheelchair?"

I had to laugh because it was true. Every gift he'd ever given me was health related. He said, "You take all the fun out of gift-giving," and for that, I apologized to him. I have always been a practical person who enjoyed receiving gifts that I would love and actually use. I guess I inherited that trait from my paternal grandmother.

One year, the family got together and bought her several gifts that we thought she would love, like bubble bath and picture frames. We even upgraded her 12 inch black and white television set to a 25 inch color set, including a remote control. We thought we had done well. By the time she opened her final gift, she instructed us to take those impractical gifts back to wherever we bought them from and come back with some gifts that she could use, like a pair of stockings that she could wear to church, a box of Kleenex to blow her nose while in church and a bag of peppermints that she could suck on in church. Ah, my grandmother was truly one of a kind and it seems I'm following in her footsteps. God rest her soul.

Thinking of my grandmother, reminds me of all the times Michael called me from the grocery store, "Babe, do you need anything?" Off the top of my head, without any hesitation, "yes, honey, pick up some Epsom Salt, so I can soak my feet and organic chamomile tea to help me relax." Poor Michael, went from isle to isle, looking for items he'd never heard of like quinoa, asking clerks where he could find currants, and probably inwardly wishing he had never called me.

What's funny is that he has not only traded in his Doritos and Cheese puffs for almonds, walnuts, goji berries, and pumpkin seeds but really enjoys them. Now, when I put together my grocery list, I take inventory of our nuts and seeds cabinet to find all the mason jars empty.

On his own, he dabs my lavender essential oil on his pillow at night and instead of taking sleep aids, he uses my liquid melatonin supplement. Honestly, at first it was a struggle, trying to convince him of mostly grocery shopping in the produce section and sticking to the perimeter isles, but when he saw how passionate I was about organics and was not willing to budge on certain products, he had no choice but to jump on board. He saw me thoroughly research the items I brought home, comparing brand to brand, reading reviews, and analyzing ingredients. He developed a level of trust in me and now, I'm happy to announce we are on one accord on our health journey together, as a team.

It's very important to have a support system, if possible. Although, if you're motivated enough, you can certainly enjoy an excellent health journey all by yourself. That's one of the main reasons I decided to become a wellness coach, so that I could be a support system and positive influence for those that don't have it but need it and passionately want it.

Ever since I was a little girl, people have always told me that they see something special in me, my passion for life. They nor I knew at the time what that passion would turn into. But, I am grateful that it was in my nature since childhood. As an adult, that passion has flourished into something beautiful, something I can't keep to myself, something I'm compelled to share. And, that's exactly what I do whenever the opportunity presents itself.

I remember, one day I went to a store in Miami to get my husband a fishing license. There was a woman standing in line before us smelling a bottle of lotion she intended to purchase. She looked back at me and extended her arm, "do you like this fragrance?" I put my nose to the nozzle and inhaled, "it's a lovely scent, but I don't use lotion. I use olive oil or coconut oil on my skin. If you can't eat it, don't put it on your skin," I advised. I could see the wheels in her head turning. After about a minute or so, she asked me to hold her place in line so she could return the lotion to its rightful place, on the shelf. She walked back smiling, "Thank you," she said. I smiled back and handed her my business card.

It's examples like this that motivates me. When I see an opportunity to make a small or large difference in someone's life and they are receptive to it, it just confirms I'm on the right track. I love helping people. I always have. I know without a shadow of a doubt, it's my calling. To be blessed to feel as much gratitude as I do on a daily basis by helping someone is a privilege and an honor. I wear my servant hat proudly. It's all I know.

3. *Ways to reduce toxins*

- Brush and floss your teeth after every meal and drink black tea for oral hygiene
- Do not eat canned foods
- Avoid plastic water bottles, Tupperware, and any other plastic laced with BPA (bisphenol A) or PVC (Polyvinyl chloride)
- Use only natural household cleaners
- Lose excess fat
- Sit less...Move more
- Do not use make-up containing phthalates, parabens
- Do not use products containing Triclosan
- Remove silver-mercury fillings from your dental work
- Stop eating pesticide-laden, genetically modified, processed foods
- Stop substance abuse
- Heal your gut
- Get enough sleep
- Drastically reduce stress levels

To enroll in the Healthy Living Program-Central Florida Operation Detox: go to healthnutsuzy.com and book your appointment.

Cleansing Diet Recipe

Kale, Pineapple and Ginger Detox Recipe

This purifying beverage contains kale to cleanse the kidneys: pineapple, which has bromelain to aid digestion; and ginger to help stimulate bile flow in your gallbladder.

Ingredients:
½ cup pineapple
2 large cucumbers
1 bunch kale without stems (4 cups chopped)
½ lemon, squeezed
¼ inch of ginger
1 bunch of mint (1/2 cup)

8.

Connecting the Dots

▼

Keep your Body strong, your Mind sharp, your Soul nourished and Spirit positive

Whether you are attempting to lose weight, quit smoking, eat healthier, combat stress or reduce your toxin levels, it all boils down to self-control. Once you've figured out what your health goals are, you must hold yourself accountable. In order for any of the strategies to work in your life, you must be disciplined to some degree to reap any benefits.

1. *How to hold yourself accountable*

a. Write up a contract with yourself

- How you will achieve your goal
- Rewards and consequences for you meeting or not meeting your goal
- Sign it to make it official
- Have a friend, family member or accountability partner witness it

b. Make it public

- Use social media to share your goals and progress
- Post your goal on Facebook

- Share weekly or monthly updates on Twitter
- Start a blog about your weight loss journey
- Keep a video diary on You Tube
- Tell a friend

c. Keep a food journal to track your progress
   If you know you have to record what you eat, you may decide against that big slice of cake or other temptation.
d. Schedule check-ins
   Have someone follow up with you daily, weekly, or monthly via phone, email, text or Facebook message. You're more likely to do something when you know someone is going to follow-up with you about it.
e. Put money on the line (you can put anything on the line, it doesn't have to be money)
   Find something that will motivate you to achieve your goals. Commit to paying a friend, family member, or coworker a designated amount of money if you don't achieve your goal.

Invest in yourself

You allow your body to function at its very best when you eat nutritious foods, exercise, get enough sleep, stress less, maintain a healthy weight and reduce toxin intake. Look at your health as an investment that you expect to yield a hefty return, which is a long healthy life.

2. What is the real root cause of disease?

I've heard it all, from:

- Inflammation
- Too many toxins
- Vitamin D deficiency

- Stress
- Emotional blockages
- Chakra imbalances
- Eating a Standard American Diet
- Not eating enough whole foods
- Mineral deficiencies
- Having a toxic gut
- Too much mucus in the body
- Having a low digestive fire
- Born with too little Jing
- Being genetically predisposed
- Loneliness

Research has indicated on the placebo effect that the power of community support is the thing that makes you healthy. Feeling lonely is the equivalent of dying a slow death. So, go be a part of something; volunteer at a nursing home facility, join your local creative writing guild or a toastmasters club. Connect with a community that can help you feel alive again.

3. Prayer v's Meditation

When asked, "Should I meditate or pray?" My answer is, both...

Prayer is seeking communication with God; whether to ask him for something, say thanks for your blessings or just be in his presence. To communicate with the creator of our universe and all of us who live in it is essential for spiritual growth and understanding, as well as healings, blessings, favor and repentance.

Meditation, on the other hand, has its perks, too. It is the most effective way to manage stress. Sitting silently, allowing God to manifest his communications through intuition or inspiration. Your mind will innately clear itself of thoughts while quieting the mind. Meditation can give you a physical and mental calm over your entire body.

RECAP: *Prayer* is speaking to God and *Meditation* is allowing the spirit of God to speak to you. They are equally important in different ways. Both prayer and meditation can give you joy and profound peace.

Prayer example: Lord, thank you for allowing me to see another day. Thank you for your loving hand of protection that surrounds me and my family. Thank you for the food on our table, the roof over our heads and the clothes on our backs. Thank you for my health and strength. I just wanted to take the first moments out of my day, before my feet even hit the ground to say, I love you and thank you, for all of the many blessings you've bestowed upon me, throughout my life. And Lord, I'm suffering with this ailment today. I ask you to touch my body in a way that only you can. Please heal me of this situation. I repent of my sins and intend to be Heaven bound and live out the rest of my days with you, in the event I've completed my earthly tasks. Amen!

Meditation example: Find a quiet, soothing environment, position yourself comfortably and focus on your breathing. Find that quiet spot within and pay attention to your body's subtle messages. With each breath, allow yourself to feel more relaxed. Imagine a golden light of healing energy, flowing through your body, slowly moving upward from your toes to the top of your head. Believe with your mind, that your body is healed of anything that ails it. Let the healing light bathe you entirely as it gently climbs higher, washing over every cell. Allow God's beautiful light to cleanse you of all negative thoughts. Trust in your body's ability to heal itself. Have faith that God wants to make you whole. Listen for his instructions by way of wisdom, intuition and inspiration. Envision yourself well and full of life. Thank your creator for the healing.

4. What is a wellness coach?

Wellness Coach:

A wellness coach will help you reach your nutrition, fitness, weight management, stress management and smoking cessation health goals by introducing you to traditional as well as alternative healing methods.

Holistic Wellness Coach:

A holistic wellness coach helps clients in the same way as a traditional wellness coach but takes it a step further by incorporating Ayurvedic principles; one of the world's oldest holistic, whole-body healing systems.

Example 1: A wellness coach may share information with a client on how to eat the appropriate amount of fruits and vegetables, of any kind.

A holistic wellness coach will consider the clients' body-type and share information that is uniquely suited to his/her specific physiology. If a client is Vata body-type, eating certain raw vegetables, for instance, could throw them out of balance, causing mood swings and other health issues.

Example 2: A wellness coach may share information with a client on how to get adequate amounts of exercise, of any kind.
A holistic wellness coach will consider a person's body-type to restore balance. If a person has a fast metabolism, lighter types of exercise will better put the body into balance, such as yoga, walking or light cycling and vice versa. If a Vata body-type performed high-intensity aerobics, the body could become imbalanced, causing unexplained health problems to develop.

Have you ever gone to the doctor complaining of an ailment and they could not find a cause for your symptoms? They take tests, and still...nothing? Many times, we experience unexplained aches and pains in our bodies that don't show up on ex-rays, or any other test. That is because, you aren't really sick. You're just out of balance.

5. Why I became a holistic wellness coach

I was born in Chicago, Illinois and raised in New Orleans, Louisiana, until Hurricane Katrina came along and destroyed the city. New Orleans is known for many wonderful things, good food being one of them. By good, I mean...tasty, spicy and just downright amazing. Unfortunately, it is also very unhealthy. The food is cooked with plenty of butter, sugar, salt, unhealthy fats and is mostly fried. It was hard for me to maintain a healthy diet while living there. A lot of my friends are now diabetic, and others have passed away due to the disease. Others have high cholesterol, high blood pressure and a host of other unfortunate health problems. I felt compelled to do something to help. I designed online health and wellness courses, put programs together, participated in health and wellness events and offered coaching sessions for free to those interested.

6. Why everyone should have a wellness coach?

Everyone could benefit from a support system, someone to help motivate and cheer you on. I find, most people's biggest challenge with making healthy lifestyle changes boils down to one simple thing...lack of discipline. That's it!

It's important to know how to exercise your discipline and increase its strength over time, instead of desperately searching for a quick fix that won't stick.

Your coach is your very own personal biggest fan, whom you can trust to sincerely want to see you succeed. A coach can look at you objectively in a way you cannot do for yourself and give you an honest assessment.

A good coach will treat you as an individual and personalize health and lifestyle plans, instead of giving you generalized information that you could find yourself on the internet.

A great coach does not have to have initials after their name but instead, help you successfully transition from willpower to discipline. Your coach will identify your strengths and weaknesses and help develop them so that you get the results you seek, and then hold you accountable to help you maintain those results.

7. Health benefits of hiring a wellness coach

- Eat healthier
- Get fit
- Relax
- Lose weight

- Quit smoking
- Set attainable goals
- Make healthy lifestyle choices
- A partner to help keep you disciplined

8. 14 Holistic healthcare Therapies

You would go to an Acupressurist if you want to receive the alternative treatment called **Acupressure;** a technique very similar to acupuncture. It's based on the concept of life energy which flows through meridians in the body. In treatment, physical pressure is applied to acupuncture points with the goal of clearing blockages in these meridians.

You should seek treatment from an Acupuncturist if you are interested in receiving the alternative therapy called **Acupuncture;** Involves pricking the skin or tissues with needles. When needles are inserted into these points, it is said that the energy flow can be brought back into proper balance. This technique is used to alleviate pain and to treat various physical, mental and emotional conditions.

You must see an Aromatherapist If you're looking to have an **Aromatherapy** treatment; a type of alternative medicine that uses essential oils and other aromatic plant compounds which are aimed at improving a person's health or mood.

Be sure to read the reviews when searching for a Chelation Therapist. **Chelation Therapy** is a medical procedure that removes heavy metals from the body and is administered under careful medical supervision.

Chiropractic is the largest alternative medical profession today. **Chiropractors** focus on diagnosis and treatment of mechanical disorders of the musculoskeletal system, especially the spine, under the belief that these disorders affect general health via the nervous system.

A Colour Therapist specializes in **Colour Therapy** (or otherwise known as Chromotherapy) which uses light in the form of color to balance energy lacking from a person's body, whether on a physical, emotional, spiritual or mental level.

A Craniosacral Therapist uses **Craniosacral Therapy;** a gentle hands-on approach, performing manipulations of the skull to release tensions deep in the body to relieve pain and dysfunction and improve whole-body health and performance.

An Herbalist practices **Herbalism;** the use of plants for medicinal purposes.

Homeopathy is the treatment of disease by minute doses of natural substances that in a healthy person would produce symptoms of disease.

A massage therapist practices **Massage Therapy;** manual manipulation of soft body tissues; muscle, connective tissue, tendons and ligaments to enhance a person's health and well-being. There are dozens of types of massage therapy.

A Naturopathic Doctor practices **Naturopathy;** the treatment of disease that avoids drugs and surgery and emphasizes the use of natural agents; such as air, water and herbs and physical means such as tissue manipulation and electrotherapy.

A Nutritionist is a person who advises on matters of food and the impact **Nutrition** has on your health.

You would go to see a Reflexologist if you were interested in having the alternative treatment **Reflexology;** involving application of pressure to the feet and hands with specific thumb, finger and hand techniques, without the use of oil or lotion. It's based on a system of zones and reflex areas that reflect an image of the body on the feet and hands with the premise that such work affects a physical change to the body.

A Reiki Practitioner practices either traditional or Christian **Reiki;** a healing technique based on the principle that a therapist can channel energy into the patient by means of touch to activate the natural healing processes of the patient's body to restore physical and emotional well-being.

About the Author

Susanna K. Green is a Certified Holistic Nutrition Professional, Reiki Master, Relaxation Massage Therapist, an Online Health & Wellness Instructor and a Certified Holistic Wellness Coach, specializing in the areas of nutrition, fitness, weight management, stress management and smoking cessation.

Susanna is the founder of the Healthy Living Program, Central Florida-Operation Detox, in Central Florida, where she resides with her husband, Michael and Toy Poodle, Laila.

www.ingramcontent.com/pod-product-compliance
Lightning Source LLC
Chambersburg PA
CBHW072237290326
41934CB00008BB/1319